This Book Belongs To:

_____

Today's Goal _____   (M) (T) (W) (T) (F) **(S) (S)**

Muscle Group Focus _____   Weight _____   Date/Time _____

Stretch ◯   Warm-Up _____

Strength Training

Exercise		Set 1	Set 2	Set 3	Set 4	Set 5	Set 6
	Reps						
	Weight						
	Reps						
	Weight						
	Reps						
	Weight						
	Reps						
	Weight						
	Reps						
	Weight						
	Reps						
	Weight						
	Reps						
	Weight						
	Reps						
	Weight						
	Reps						
	Weight						
	Reps						
	Weight						

Cardio

Exercise	Calories	Distance	Time

Water Intake _____

Cooldown _____

Feeling ☆ ☆ ☆ ☆ ☆

Notes

Today's Goal _____ (M) (T) (W) (T) (F) **(S) (S)**

Muscle Group Focus _____   Weight _____   Date/Time _____

Stretch ◯   Warm-Up _____

Strength Training

Exercise		Set 1	Set 2	Set 3	Set 4	Set 5	Set 6
	Reps						
	Weight						
	Reps						
	Weight						
	Reps						
	Weight						
	Reps						
	Weight						
	Reps						
	Weight						
	Reps						
	Weight						
	Reps						
	Weight						
	Reps						
	Weight						
	Reps						
	Weight						
	Reps						
	Weight						

Cardio

Exercise	Calories	Distance	Time

Water Intake _____

Cooldown _____

Feeling ☆ ☆ ☆ ☆ ☆

Notes

Today's Goal _____   (M) (T) (W) (T) (F) **(S) (S)**

Muscle Group Focus _____   Weight _____   Date/Time _____

Stretch ◯   Warm-Up _____

Strength Training

Exercise		Set 1	Set 2	Set 3	Set 4	Set 5	Set 6
	Reps						
	Weight						
	Reps						
	Weight						
	Reps						
	Weight						
	Reps						
	Weight						
	Reps						
	Weight						
	Reps						
	Weight						
	Reps						
	Weight						
	Reps						
	Weight						
	Reps						
	Weight						
	Reps						
	Weight						

Cardio

Exercise	Calories	Distance	Time

Water Intake _____

Cooldown _____

Feeling ☆ ☆ ☆ ☆ ☆

Notes

Today's Goal

(M) (T) (W) (T) (F) **(S) (S)**

Muscle Group Focus _____   Weight _____   Date/Time _____

Stretch ○   Warm-Up _____

Strength Training

Exercise		Set 1	Set 2	Set 3	Set 4	Set 5	Set 6
	Reps						
	Weight						
	Reps						
	Weight						
	Reps						
	Weight						
	Reps						
	Weight						
	Reps						
	Weight						
	Reps						
	Weight						
	Reps						
	Weight						
	Reps						
	Weight						
	Reps						
	Weight						

Cardio

Exercise	Calories	Distance	Time

Water Intake _____

Cooldown _____

Feeling ☆ ☆ ☆ ☆ ☆

Notes

Today's Goal

(M) (T) (W) (T) (F) **(S) (S)**

Muscle Group Focus _____   Weight _____   Date/Time _____

Stretch ◯   Warm-Up _____

Strength Training

Exercise		Set 1	Set 2	Set 3	Set 4	Set 5	Set 6
	Reps						
	Weight						
	Reps						
	Weight						
	Reps						
	Weight						
	Reps						
	Weight						
	Reps						
	Weight						
	Reps						
	Weight						
	Reps						
	Weight						
	Reps						
	Weight						
	Reps						
	Weight						
	Reps						
	Weight						

Cardio

Exercise	Calories	Distance	Time

Water Intake _____

Cooldown _____

Feeling ☆ ☆ ☆ ☆ ☆

Notes

Today's Goal _____ Ⓜ Ⓣ Ⓦ Ⓣ Ⓕ ●S ●S

Muscle Group Focus _____ Weight _____ Date/Time _____

Stretch ◯   Warm-Up _____

Strength Training

Exercise		Set 1	Set 2	Set 3	Set 4	Set 5	Set 6
	Reps						
	Weight						
	Reps						
	Weight						
	Reps						
	Weight						
	Reps						
	Weight						
	Reps						
	Weight						
	Reps						
	Weight						
	Reps						
	Weight						
	Reps						
	Weight						
	Reps						
	Weight						
	Reps						
	Weight						

Cardio

Exercise	Calories	Distance	Time

Water Intake _____

Cooldown _____

Feeling ☆ ☆ ☆ ☆ ☆

Notes

Today's Goal _____   (M) (T) (W) (T) (F) **(S) (S)**

Muscle Group Focus _____   Weight _____   Date/Time _____

Stretch ○   Warm-Up _____

Strength Training

Exercise		Set 1	Set 2	Set 3	Set 4	Set 5	Set 6
	Reps						
	Weight						
	Reps						
	Weight						
	Reps						
	Weight						
	Reps						
	Weight						
	Reps						
	Weight						
	Reps						
	Weight						
	Reps						
	Weight						
	Reps						
	Weight						
	Reps						
	Weight						
	Reps						
	Weight						

Cardio

Exercise	Calories	Distance	Time

Water Intake _____

Cooldown _____

Feeling ☆ ☆ ☆ ☆ ☆

Notes

Today's Goal _____   (M) (T) (W) (T) (F) **(S) (S)**

Muscle Group Focus _____   Weight _____   Date/Time _____

Stretch ○   Warm-Up _____

Strength Training

Exercise		Set 1	Set 2	Set 3	Set 4	Set 5	Set 6
	Reps						
	Weight						
	Reps						
	Weight						
	Reps						
	Weight						
	Reps						
	Weight						
	Reps						
	Weight						
	Reps						
	Weight						
	Reps						
	Weight						
	Reps						
	Weight						
	Reps						
	Weight						
	Reps						
	Weight						

Cardio

Exercise	Calories	Distance	Time

Water Intake _____

Cooldown _____

Feeling ☆ ☆ ☆ ☆ ☆

Notes

Today's Goal _____   (M) (T) (W) (T) (F) **(S) (S)**

Muscle Group Focus _____   Weight _____   Date/Time _____

Stretch ○   Warm-Up _____

Strength Training

Exercise		Set 1	Set 2	Set 3	Set 4	Set 5	Set 6
	Reps						
	Weight						
	Reps						
	Weight						
	Reps						
	Weight						
	Reps						
	Weight						
	Reps						
	Weight						
	Reps						
	Weight						
	Reps						
	Weight						
	Reps						
	Weight						
	Reps						
	Weight						
	Reps						
	Weight						

Cardio

Exercise	Calories	Distance	Time

Water Intake _____

Cooldown _____

Feeling ☆ ☆ ☆ ☆ ☆

Notes

Today's Goal

(M) (T) (W) (T) (F) (S) (S)

Muscle Group Focus _____   Weight _____   Date/Time _____

Stretch ◯   Warm-Up _____

Strength Training

Exercise		Set 1	Set 2	Set 3	Set 4	Set 5	Set 6
	Reps						
	Weight						
	Reps						
	Weight						
	Reps						
	Weight						
	Reps						
	Weight						
	Reps						
	Weight						
	Reps						
	Weight						
	Reps						
	Weight						
	Reps						
	Weight						
	Reps						
	Weight						
	Reps						
	Weight						

Cardio

Exercise	Calories	Distance	Time

Water Intake _____

Cooldown _____

Feeling ☆ ☆ ☆ ☆ ☆

Notes

Today's Goal _____ (M) (T) (W) (T) (F) ●S ●S

Muscle Group Focus _____   Weight _____   Date/Time _____

Stretch ○   Warm-Up _____

Strength Training

Exercise		Set 1	Set 2	Set 3	Set 4	Set 5	Set 6
	Reps						
	Weight						
	Reps						
	Weight						
	Reps						
	Weight						
	Reps						
	Weight						
	Reps						
	Weight						
	Reps						
	Weight						
	Reps						
	Weight						
	Reps						
	Weight						
	Reps						
	Weight						
	Reps						
	Weight						

Cardio

Exercise	Calories	Distance	Time

Water Intake _____

Cooldown _____

Feeling ☆ ☆ ☆ ☆ ☆

Notes

Today's Goal _____   Ⓜ Ⓣ Ⓦ Ⓣ Ⓕ ●S ●S

Muscle Group Focus _____   Weight _____   Date/Time _____

Stretch ◯   Warm-Up _____

Strength Training

Exercise		Set 1	Set 2	Set 3	Set 4	Set 5	Set 6
	Reps						
	Weight						
	Reps						
	Weight						
	Reps						
	Weight						
	Reps						
	Weight						
	Reps						
	Weight						
	Reps						
	Weight						
	Reps						
	Weight						
	Reps						
	Weight						
	Reps						
	Weight						
	Reps						
	Weight						

Cardio

Exercise	Calories	Distance	Time

Water Intake _____

Cooldown _____

Feeling ☆ ☆ ☆ ☆ ☆

Notes

Today's Goal _____   (M) (T) (W) (T) (F) (S) (S)

Muscle Group Focus _____   Weight _____   Date/Time _____

Stretch ○   Warm-Up _____

Strength Training

Exercise		Set 1	Set 2	Set 3	Set 4	Set 5	Set 6
	Reps						
	Weight						
	Reps						
	Weight						
	Reps						
	Weight						
	Reps						
	Weight						
	Reps						
	Weight						
	Reps						
	Weight						
	Reps						
	Weight						
	Reps						
	Weight						
	Reps						
	Weight						
	Reps						
	Weight						

Cardio

Exercise	Calories	Distance	Time

Water Intake _____

Cooldown _____

Feeling ☆ ☆ ☆ ☆ ☆

Notes

Today's Goal _____   (M) (T) (W) (T) (F) ●S ●S

Muscle Group Focus _____   Weight _____   Date/Time _____

Stretch ◯   Warm-Up _____

Strength Training

Exercise		Set 1	Set 2	Set 3	Set 4	Set 5	Set 6
	Reps						
	Weight						
	Reps						
	Weight						
	Reps						
	Weight						
	Reps						
	Weight						
	Reps						
	Weight						
	Reps						
	Weight						
	Reps						
	Weight						
	Reps						
	Weight						
	Reps						
	Weight						
	Reps						
	Weight						

Cardio

Exercise	Calories	Distance	Time

Water Intake _____

Cooldown _____

Feeling ☆ ☆ ☆ ☆ ☆

Notes

Today's Goal _____ (M) (T) (W) (T) (F) ●S ●S

Muscle Group Focus _____   Weight _____   Date/Time _____

Stretch ○   Warm-Up _____

Strength Training

Exercise		Set 1	Set 2	Set 3	Set 4	Set 5	Set 6
	Reps						
	Weight						
	Reps						
	Weight						
	Reps						
	Weight						
	Reps						
	Weight						
	Reps						
	Weight						
	Reps						
	Weight						
	Reps						
	Weight						
	Reps						
	Weight						
	Reps						
	Weight						
	Reps						
	Weight						

Cardio

Exercise	Calories	Distance	Time

Water Intake _____

Cooldown _____

Feeling ☆ ☆ ☆ ☆ ☆

Notes

Today's Goal _____   (M) (T) (W) (T) (F) **S** **S**

Muscle Group Focus _____   Weight _____   Date/Time _____

Stretch ○   Warm-Up _____

Strength Training

Exercise		Set 1	Set 2	Set 3	Set 4	Set 5	Set 6
	Reps						
	Weight						
	Reps						
	Weight						
	Reps						
	Weight						
	Reps						
	Weight						
	Reps						
	Weight						
	Reps						
	Weight						
	Reps						
	Weight						
	Reps						
	Weight						
	Reps						
	Weight						
	Reps						
	Weight						

Cardio

Exercise	Calories	Distance	Time

Water Intake _____

Cooldown _____

Feeling ☆ ☆ ☆ ☆ ☆

Notes

Today's Goal _____   (M) (T) (W) (T) (F) ●S ●S

Muscle Group Focus _____   Weight _____   Date/Time _____

Stretch ○   Warm-Up _____

Strength Training

Exercise		Set 1	Set 2	Set 3	Set 4	Set 5	Set 6
	Reps						
	Weight						
	Reps						
	Weight						
	Reps						
	Weight						
	Reps						
	Weight						
	Reps						
	Weight						
	Reps						
	Weight						
	Reps						
	Weight						
	Reps						
	Weight						
	Reps						
	Weight						
	Reps						
	Weight						

Cardio

Exercise	Calories	Distance	Time

Water Intake _____

Cooldown _____

Feeling ☆ ☆ ☆ ☆ ☆

Notes

Today's Goal _____ (M) (T) (W) (T) (F) **(S) (S)**

Muscle Group Focus _____   Weight _____   Date/Time _____

Stretch ○   Warm-Up _____

Strength Training

Exercise		Set 1	Set 2	Set 3	Set 4	Set 5	Set 6
	Reps						
	Weight						
	Reps						
	Weight						
	Reps						
	Weight						
	Reps						
	Weight						
	Reps						
	Weight						
	Reps						
	Weight						
	Reps						
	Weight						
	Reps						
	Weight						
	Reps						
	Weight						
	Reps						
	Weight						

Cardio

Exercise		Calories	Distance	Time

Water Intake _____

Cooldown _____

Feeling ☆ ☆ ☆ ☆ ☆

Notes

Today's Goal _____   (M) (T) (W) (T) (F) **(S) (S)**

Muscle Group Focus _____   Weight _____   Date/Time _____

Stretch ◯   Warm-Up _____

Strength Training

Exercise		Set 1	Set 2	Set 3	Set 4	Set 5	Set 6
	Reps						
	Weight						
	Reps						
	Weight						
	Reps						
	Weight						
	Reps						
	Weight						
	Reps						
	Weight						
	Reps						
	Weight						
	Reps						
	Weight						
	Reps						
	Weight						
	Reps						
	Weight						
	Reps						
	Weight						

Cardio

Exercise	Calories	Distance	Time

Water Intake _____

Cooldown _____

Feeling ☆ ☆ ☆ ☆ ☆

Notes

Today's Goal _____   (M) (T) (W) (T) (F) ●S ●S

Muscle Group Focus _____   Weight _____   Date/Time _____

Stretch ○   Warm-Up _____

Strength Training

Exercise		Set 1	Set 2	Set 3	Set 4	Set 5	Set 6
	Reps						
	Weight						
	Reps						
	Weight						
	Reps						
	Weight						
	Reps						
	Weight						
	Reps						
	Weight						
	Reps						
	Weight						
	Reps						
	Weight						
	Reps						
	Weight						
	Reps						
	Weight						
	Reps						
	Weight						

Cardio

Exercise	Calories	Distance	Time

Water Intake _____

Cooldown _____

Feeling ☆ ☆ ☆ ☆ ☆

Notes

Today's Goal _____   Ⓜ Ⓣ Ⓦ Ⓣ Ⓕ ● ●

Muscle Group Focus _____   Weight _____   Date/Time _____

Stretch ○   Warm-Up _____

Strength Training

Exercise		Set 1	Set 2	Set 3	Set 4	Set 5	Set 6
	Reps						
	Weight						
	Reps						
	Weight						
	Reps						
	Weight						
	Reps						
	Weight						
	Reps						
	Weight						
	Reps						
	Weight						
	Reps						
	Weight						
	Reps						
	Weight						
	Reps						
	Weight						
	Reps						
	Weight						

Cardio

Exercise	Calories	Distance	Time

Water Intake _____

Cooldown _____

Feeling ☆ ☆ ☆ ☆ ☆

Notes

Today's Goal _____   (M) (T) (W) (T) (F) ●S ●S

Muscle Group Focus _____   Weight _____   Date/Time _____

Stretch ○   Warm-Up _____

Strength Training

Exercise		Set 1	Set 2	Set 3	Set 4	Set 5	Set 6
	Reps						
	Weight						
	Reps						
	Weight						
	Reps						
	Weight						
	Reps						
	Weight						
	Reps						
	Weight						
	Reps						
	Weight						
	Reps						
	Weight						
	Reps						
	Weight						
	Reps						
	Weight						
	Reps						
	Weight						

Cardio

Exercise	Calories	Distance	Time

Water Intake _____

Cooldown _____

Feeling ☆ ☆ ☆ ☆ ☆

Notes

Today's Goal _____   (M) (T) (W) (T) (F) **(S) (S)**

Muscle Group Focus _____   Weight _____   Date/Time _____

Stretch ◯   Warm-Up _____

Strength Training

Exercise		Set 1	Set 2	Set 3	Set 4	Set 5	Set 6
	Reps						
	Weight						
	Reps						
	Weight						
	Reps						
	Weight						
	Reps						
	Weight						
	Reps						
	Weight						
	Reps						
	Weight						
	Reps						
	Weight						
	Reps						
	Weight						
	Reps						
	Weight						
	Reps						
	Weight						

Cardio

Exercise	Calories	Distance	Time

Water Intake _____

Cooldown _____

Feeling ☆ ☆ ☆ ☆ ☆

Notes

Today's Goal

(M) (T) (W) (T) (F) **(S) (S)**

Muscle Group Focus _____ Weight _____ Date/Time _____

Stretch ○   Warm-Up _____

Strength Training

Exercise		Set 1	Set 2	Set 3	Set 4	Set 5	Set 6
	Reps						
	Weight						
	Reps						
	Weight						
	Reps						
	Weight						
	Reps						
	Weight						
	Reps						
	Weight						
	Reps						
	Weight						
	Reps						
	Weight						
	Reps						
	Weight						
	Reps						
	Weight						
	Reps						
	Weight						

Cardio

Exercise		Calories	Distance	Time

Water Intake _____

Cooldown _____

Feeling ☆ ☆ ☆ ☆ ☆

Notes

Today's Goal _____   M T W T F **S** **S**

Muscle Group Focus _____ Weight _____ Date/Time _____

Stretch ◯   Warm-Up _____

Strength Training

Exercise		Set 1	Set 2	Set 3	Set 4	Set 5	Set 6
	Reps						
	Weight						
	Reps						
	Weight						
	Reps						
	Weight						
	Reps						
	Weight						
	Reps						
	Weight						
	Reps						
	Weight						
	Reps						
	Weight						
	Reps						
	Weight						
	Reps						
	Weight						

Cardio

Exercise	Calories	Distance	Time

Water Intake _____

Cooldown _____

Feeling ☆ ☆ ☆ ☆ ☆

Notes

Today's Goal _____   (M) (T) (W) (T) (F) **(S) (S)**

Muscle Group Focus _____   Weight _____   Date/Time _____

Stretch ○   Warm-Up _____

Strength Training

Exercise		Set 1	Set 2	Set 3	Set 4	Set 5	Set 6
	Reps						
	Weight						
	Reps						
	Weight						
	Reps						
	Weight						
	Reps						
	Weight						
	Reps						
	Weight						
	Reps						
	Weight						
	Reps						
	Weight						
	Reps						
	Weight						
	Reps						
	Weight						
	Reps						
	Weight						

Cardio

Exercise	Calories	Distance	Time

Water Intake _____

Cooldown _____

Feeling ☆ ☆ ☆ ☆ ☆

Notes

Today's Goal _____   (M) (T) (W) (T) (F) ●S ●S

Muscle Group Focus _____   Weight _____   Date/Time _____

Stretch ◯   Warm-Up _____

Strength Training

Exercise		Set 1	Set 2	Set 3	Set 4	Set 5	Set 6
	Reps						
	Weight						
	Reps						
	Weight						
	Reps						
	Weight						
	Reps						
	Weight						
	Reps						
	Weight						
	Reps						
	Weight						
	Reps						
	Weight						
	Reps						
	Weight						
	Reps						
	Weight						
	Reps						
	Weight						

Cardio

Exercise	Calories	Distance	Time

Water Intake _____

Cooldown _____

Feeling ☆ ☆ ☆ ☆ ☆

Notes

Today's Goal _____   (M) (T) (W) (T) (F) ●S ●S

Muscle Group Focus _____   Weight _____   Date/Time _____

Stretch ○   Warm-Up _____

Strength Training

Exercise		Set 1	Set 2	Set 3	Set 4	Set 5	Set 6
	Reps						
	Weight						
	Reps						
	Weight						
	Reps						
	Weight						
	Reps						
	Weight						
	Reps						
	Weight						
	Reps						
	Weight						
	Reps						
	Weight						
	Reps						
	Weight						
	Reps						
	Weight						
	Reps						
	Weight						

Cardio

Exercise	Calories	Distance	Time

Water Intake _____

Cooldown _____

Feeling ☆ ☆ ☆ ☆ ☆

Notes

Today's Goal _____   (M) (T) (W) (T) (F) **(S) (S)**

Muscle Group Focus _____   Weight _____   Date/Time _____

Stretch ◯   Warm-Up _____

Strength Training

Exercise		Set 1	Set 2	Set 3	Set 4	Set 5	Set 6
	Reps						
	Weight						
	Reps						
	Weight						
	Reps						
	Weight						
	Reps						
	Weight						
	Reps						
	Weight						
	Reps						
	Weight						
	Reps						
	Weight						
	Reps						
	Weight						
	Reps						
	Weight						
	Reps						
	Weight						

Cardio

Exercise	Calories	Distance	Time

Water Intake _____

Cooldown _____

Feeling ☆ ☆ ☆ ☆ ☆

Notes

Today's Goal _____   (M) (T) (W) (T) (F) **(S) (S)**

Muscle Group Focus _____   Weight _____   Date/Time _____

Stretch ◯   Warm-Up _____

Strength Training

Exercise		Set 1	Set 2	Set 3	Set 4	Set 5	Set 6
	Reps						
	Weight						
	Reps						
	Weight						
	Reps						
	Weight						
	Reps						
	Weight						
	Reps						
	Weight						
	Reps						
	Weight						
	Reps						
	Weight						
	Reps						
	Weight						
	Reps						
	Weight						

Cardio

Exercise		Calories	Distance	Time

Water Intake _____

Cooldown _____

Feeling ☆ ☆ ☆ ☆ ☆

Notes

Today's Goal _____   (M) (T) (W) (T) (F) **(S) (S)**

Muscle Group Focus _____   Weight _____   Date/Time _____

Stretch ○   Warm-Up _____

Strength Training

Exercise		Set 1	Set 2	Set 3	Set 4	Set 5	Set 6
	Reps						
	Weight						
	Reps						
	Weight						
	Reps						
	Weight						
	Reps						
	Weight						
	Reps						
	Weight						
	Reps						
	Weight						
	Reps						
	Weight						
	Reps						
	Weight						
	Reps						
	Weight						
	Reps						
	Weight						

Cardio

Exercise	Calories	Distance	Time

Water Intake _____

Cooldown _____

Feeling ☆ ☆ ☆ ☆ ☆

Notes

Today's Goal _____   (M) (T) (W) (T) (F) **(S) (S)**

Muscle Group Focus _____   Weight _____   Date/Time _____

Stretch ○   Warm-Up _____

Strength Training

Exercise		Set 1	Set 2	Set 3	Set 4	Set 5	Set 6
	Reps						
	Weight						
	Reps						
	Weight						
	Reps						
	Weight						
	Reps						
	Weight						
	Reps						
	Weight						
	Reps						
	Weight						
	Reps						
	Weight						
	Reps						
	Weight						
	Reps						
	Weight						
	Reps						
	Weight						

Cardio

Exercise	Calories	Distance	Time

Water Intake _____

Cooldown _____

Feeling ☆ ☆ ☆ ☆ ☆

Notes

Today's Goal _____   (M) (T) (W) (T) (F) (S) (S)

Muscle Group Focus _____   Weight _____   Date/Time _____

Stretch ○   Warm-Up _____

Strength Training

Exercise		Set 1	Set 2	Set 3	Set 4	Set 5	Set 6
	Reps						
	Weight						
	Reps						
	Weight						
	Reps						
	Weight						
	Reps						
	Weight						
	Reps						
	Weight						
	Reps						
	Weight						
	Reps						
	Weight						
	Reps						
	Weight						
	Reps						
	Weight						
	Reps						
	Weight						

Cardio

Exercise	Calories	Distance	Time

Water Intake _____

Cooldown _____

Feeling ☆ ☆ ☆ ☆ ☆

Notes

Today's Goal _____   (M) (T) (W) (T) (F) ●S ●S

Muscle Group Focus _____   Weight _____   Date/Time _____

Stretch ○   Warm-Up _____

Strength Training

Exercise		Set 1	Set 2	Set 3	Set 4	Set 5	Set 6
	Reps						
	Weight						
	Reps						
	Weight						
	Reps						
	Weight						
	Reps						
	Weight						
	Reps						
	Weight						
	Reps						
	Weight						
	Reps						
	Weight						
	Reps						
	Weight						
	Reps						
	Weight						
	Reps						
	Weight						

Cardio

Exercise	Calories	Distance	Time

Water Intake _____

Cooldown _____

Feeling ☆ ☆ ☆ ☆ ☆

Notes

Today's Goal _____   (M) (T) (W) (T) (F) **(S) (S)**

Muscle Group Focus _____   Weight _____   Date/Time _____

Stretch ◯   Warm-Up _____

Strength Training

Exercise		Set 1	Set 2	Set 3	Set 4	Set 5	Set 6
	Reps						
	Weight						
	Reps						
	Weight						
	Reps						
	Weight						
	Reps						
	Weight						
	Reps						
	Weight						
	Reps						
	Weight						
	Reps						
	Weight						
	Reps						
	Weight						
	Reps						
	Weight						
	Reps						
	Weight						

Cardio

Exercise	Calories	Distance	Time

Water Intake _____

Cooldown _____

Feeling ☆ ☆ ☆ ☆ ☆

Notes

Today's Goal _____   Ⓜ Ⓣ Ⓦ Ⓣ Ⓕ **S** **S**

Muscle Group Focus _____   Weight _____   Date/Time _____

Stretch ◯   Warm-Up _____

Strength Training

Exercise		Set 1	Set 2	Set 3	Set 4	Set 5	Set 6
	Reps						
	Weight						
	Reps						
	Weight						
	Reps						
	Weight						
	Reps						
	Weight						
	Reps						
	Weight						
	Reps						
	Weight						
	Reps						
	Weight						
	Reps						
	Weight						
	Reps						
	Weight						
	Reps						
	Weight						

Cardio

Exercise	Calories	Distance	Time

Water Intake _____

Cooldown _____

Feeling ☆ ☆ ☆ ☆ ☆

Notes

Today's Goal _____   (M) (T) (W) (T) (F) (S) (S)

Muscle Group Focus _____   Weight _____   Date/Time _____

Stretch ○   Warm-Up _____

Strength Training

Exercise		Set 1	Set 2	Set 3	Set 4	Set 5	Set 6
	Reps						
	Weight						
	Reps						
	Weight						
	Reps						
	Weight						
	Reps						
	Weight						
	Reps						
	Weight						
	Reps						
	Weight						
	Reps						
	Weight						
	Reps						
	Weight						
	Reps						
	Weight						
	Reps						
	Weight						

Cardio

Exercise	Calories	Distance	Time

Water Intake _____

Cooldown _____

Feeling ☆ ☆ ☆ ☆ ☆

Notes

Today's Goal _____   Ⓜ Ⓣ Ⓦ Ⓣ Ⓕ ●S ●S

Muscle Group Focus _____   Weight _____   Date/Time _____

Stretch ○   Warm-Up _____

Strength Training

Exercise		Set 1	Set 2	Set 3	Set 4	Set 5	Set 6
	Reps						
	Weight						
	Reps						
	Weight						
	Reps						
	Weight						
	Reps						
	Weight						
	Reps						
	Weight						
	Reps						
	Weight						
	Reps						
	Weight						
	Reps						
	Weight						
	Reps						
	Weight						
	Reps						
	Weight						

Cardio

Exercise	Calories	Distance	Time

Water Intake _____

Cooldown _____

Feeling ☆ ☆ ☆ ☆ ☆

Notes

Today's Goal _____   Ⓜ Ⓣ Ⓦ Ⓣ Ⓕ ●S ●S

Muscle Group Focus _____   Weight _____   Date/Time _____

Stretch ○   Warm-Up _____

Strength Training

Exercise		Set 1	Set 2	Set 3	Set 4	Set 5	Set 6
	Reps						
	Weight						
	Reps						
	Weight						
	Reps						
	Weight						
	Reps						
	Weight						
	Reps						
	Weight						
	Reps						
	Weight						
	Reps						
	Weight						
	Reps						
	Weight						
	Reps						
	Weight						
	Reps						
	Weight						

Cardio

Exercise		Calories	Distance	Time

Water Intake _____

Cooldown _____

Feeling ☆ ☆ ☆ ☆ ☆

Notes

Today's Goal _____   Ⓜ Ⓣ Ⓦ Ⓣ Ⓕ ●S ●S

Muscle Group Focus _____   Weight _____   Date/Time _____

Stretch ○   Warm-Up _____

Strength Training

Exercise		Set 1	Set 2	Set 3	Set 4	Set 5	Set 6
	Reps						
	Weight						
	Reps						
	Weight						
	Reps						
	Weight						
	Reps						
	Weight						
	Reps						
	Weight						
	Reps						
	Weight						
	Reps						
	Weight						
	Reps						
	Weight						
	Reps						
	Weight						
	Reps						
	Weight						

Cardio

Exercise	Calories	Distance	Time

Water Intake _____

Cooldown _____

Feeling ☆☆☆☆☆

Notes

Today's Goal _____   (M) (T) (W) (T) (F) ●S ●S

Muscle Group Focus _____   Weight _____   Date/Time _____

Stretch ○   Warm-Up _____

Strength Training

Exercise		Set 1	Set 2	Set 3	Set 4	Set 5	Set 6
	Reps						
	Weight						
	Reps						
	Weight						
	Reps						
	Weight						
	Reps						
	Weight						
	Reps						
	Weight						
	Reps						
	Weight						
	Reps						
	Weight						
	Reps						
	Weight						
	Reps						
	Weight						
	Reps						
	Weight						

Cardio

Exercise	Calories	Distance	Time

Water Intake _____

Cooldown _____

Feeling ☆ ☆ ☆ ☆ ☆

Notes

Today's Goal _____ (M) (T) (W) (T) (F) **(S) (S)**

Muscle Group Focus _____   Weight _____   Date/Time _____

Stretch ○   Warm-Up _____

Strength Training

Exercise		Set 1	Set 2	Set 3	Set 4	Set 5	Set 6
	Reps						
	Weight						
	Reps						
	Weight						
	Reps						
	Weight						
	Reps						
	Weight						
	Reps						
	Weight						
	Reps						
	Weight						
	Reps						
	Weight						
	Reps						
	Weight						
	Reps						
	Weight						
	Reps						
	Weight						

Cardio

Exercise	Calories	Distance	Time

Water Intake _____

Cooldown _____

Feeling ☆ ☆ ☆ ☆ ☆

Notes

Today's Goal

(M) (T) (W) (T) (F) **(S) (S)**

Muscle Group Focus _____   Weight _____   Date/Time _____

Stretch ○   Warm-Up _____

Strength Training

Exercise		Set 1	Set 2	Set 3	Set 4	Set 5	Set 6
	Reps						
	Weight						
	Reps						
	Weight						
	Reps						
	Weight						
	Reps						
	Weight						
	Reps						
	Weight						
	Reps						
	Weight						
	Reps						
	Weight						
	Reps						
	Weight						
	Reps						
	Weight						
	Reps						
	Weight						

Cardio

Exercise	Calories	Distance	Time

Water Intake _____

Cooldown _____

Feeling ☆ ☆ ☆ ☆ ☆

Notes

Today's Goal _____   (M) (T) (W) (T) (F) **S** **S**

Muscle Group Focus _____   Weight _____   Date/Time _____

Stretch ○   Warm-Up _____

Strength Training

Exercise		Set 1	Set 2	Set 3	Set 4	Set 5	Set 6
	Reps						
	Weight						
	Reps						
	Weight						
	Reps						
	Weight						
	Reps						
	Weight						
	Reps						
	Weight						
	Reps						
	Weight						
	Reps						
	Weight						
	Reps						
	Weight						
	Reps						
	Weight						
	Reps						
	Weight						

Cardio

Exercise	Calories	Distance	Time

Water Intake _____

Cooldown _____

Feeling ☆ ☆ ☆ ☆ ☆

Notes

Today's Goal _____   (M) (T) (W) (T) (F) ● ●

Muscle Group Focus _____   Weight _____   Date/Time _____

Stretch ○   Warm-Up _____

Strength Training

Exercise		Set 1	Set 2	Set 3	Set 4	Set 5	Set 6
	Reps						
	Weight						
	Reps						
	Weight						
	Reps						
	Weight						
	Reps						
	Weight						
	Reps						
	Weight						
	Reps						
	Weight						
	Reps						
	Weight						
	Reps						
	Weight						
	Reps						
	Weight						
	Reps						
	Weight						

Cardio

Exercise	Calories	Distance	Time

Water Intake _____

Cooldown _____

Feeling ☆ ☆ ☆ ☆ ☆

Notes

Today's Goal

(M) (T) (W) (T) (F) **(S)** **(S)**

Muscle Group Focus _____   Weight _____   Date/Time _____

Stretch ○   Warm-Up _____

Strength Training

Exercise		Set 1	Set 2	Set 3	Set 4	Set 5	Set 6
	Reps						
	Weight						
	Reps						
	Weight						
	Reps						
	Weight						
	Reps						
	Weight						
	Reps						
	Weight						
	Reps						
	Weight						
	Reps						
	Weight						
	Reps						
	Weight						
	Reps						
	Weight						
	Reps						
	Weight						

Cardio

Exercise	Calories	Distance	Time

Water Intake _____

Cooldown _____

Feeling ☆☆☆☆☆

Notes

Today's Goal _____   (M) (T) (W) (T) (F) ● ●

Muscle Group Focus _____   Weight _____   Date/Time _____

Stretch ○   Warm-Up _____

Strength Training

Exercise		Set 1	Set 2	Set 3	Set 4	Set 5	Set 6
	Reps						
	Weight						
	Reps						
	Weight						
	Reps						
	Weight						
	Reps						
	Weight						
	Reps						
	Weight						
	Reps						
	Weight						
	Reps						
	Weight						
	Reps						
	Weight						
	Reps						
	Weight						
	Reps						
	Weight						

Cardio

Exercise	Calories	Distance	Time

Water Intake _____

Cooldown _____

Feeling ☆ ☆ ☆ ☆ ☆

Notes

Today's Goal _____   Ⓜ Ⓣ Ⓦ Ⓣ Ⓕ ● ●

Muscle Group Focus _____   Weight _____   Date/Time _____

Stretch ○   Warm-Up _____

Strength Training

Exercise		Set 1	Set 2	Set 3	Set 4	Set 5	Set 6
	Reps						
	Weight						
	Reps						
	Weight						
	Reps						
	Weight						
	Reps						
	Weight						
	Reps						
	Weight						
	Reps						
	Weight						
	Reps						
	Weight						
	Reps						
	Weight						
	Reps						
	Weight						
	Reps						
	Weight						

Cardio

Exercise	Calories	Distance	Time

Water Intake _____

Cooldown _____

Feeling ☆ ☆ ☆ ☆ ☆

Notes

Today's Goal _____   (M) (T) (W) (T) (F) **(S) (S)**

Muscle Group Focus _____   Weight _____   Date/Time _____

Stretch ○   Warm-Up _____

Strength Training

Exercise		Set 1	Set 2	Set 3	Set 4	Set 5	Set 6
	Reps						
	Weight						
	Reps						
	Weight						
	Reps						
	Weight						
	Reps						
	Weight						
	Reps						
	Weight						
	Reps						
	Weight						
	Reps						
	Weight						
	Reps						
	Weight						
	Reps						
	Weight						
	Reps						
	Weight						

Cardio

Exercise	Calories	Distance	Time

Water Intake _____

Cooldown _____

Feeling ☆ ☆ ☆ ☆ ☆

Notes

Today's Goal _____   (M) (T) (W) (T) (F) ● ●

Muscle Group Focus _____   Weight _____   Date/Time _____

Stretch ○   Warm-Up _____

Strength Training

Exercise		Set 1	Set 2	Set 3	Set 4	Set 5	Set 6
	Reps						
	Weight						
	Reps						
	Weight						
	Reps						
	Weight						
	Reps						
	Weight						
	Reps						
	Weight						
	Reps						
	Weight						
	Reps						
	Weight						
	Reps						
	Weight						
	Reps						
	Weight						
	Reps						
	Weight						

Cardio

Exercise	Calories	Distance	Time

Water Intake _____

Cooldown _____

Feeling ☆ ☆ ☆ ☆ ☆

Notes

Today's Goal _____ (M) (T) (W) (T) (F) **(S) (S)**

Muscle Group Focus _____   Weight _____   Date/Time _____

Stretch ○   Warm-Up _____

Strength Training

Exercise		Set 1	Set 2	Set 3	Set 4	Set 5	Set 6
	Reps						
	Weight						
	Reps						
	Weight						
	Reps						
	Weight						
	Reps						
	Weight						
	Reps						
	Weight						
	Reps						
	Weight						
	Reps						
	Weight						
	Reps						
	Weight						
	Reps						
	Weight						
	Reps						
	Weight						

Cardio

Exercise	Calories	Distance	Time

Water Intake _____

Cooldown _____

Feeling ☆ ☆ ☆ ☆ ☆

Notes

Today's Goal _____   (M) (T) (W) (T) (F) **(S) (S)**

Muscle Group Focus _____   Weight _____   Date/Time _____

Stretch ◯   Warm-Up _____

Strength Training

Exercise		Set 1	Set 2	Set 3	Set 4	Set 5	Set 6
	Reps						
	Weight						
	Reps						
	Weight						
	Reps						
	Weight						
	Reps						
	Weight						
	Reps						
	Weight						
	Reps						
	Weight						
	Reps						
	Weight						
	Reps						
	Weight						
	Reps						
	Weight						
	Reps						
	Weight						

Cardio

Exercise	Calories	Distance	Time

Water Intake _____

Cooldown _____

Feeling ☆ ☆ ☆ ☆ ☆

Notes

Today's Goal ⟶ _____   (M) (T) (W) (T) (F) **(S) (S)**

Muscle Group Focus _____   Weight _____   Date/Time _____

Stretch ○   Warm-Up _____

Strength Training

Exercise		Set 1	Set 2	Set 3	Set 4	Set 5	Set 6
	Reps						
	Weight						
	Reps						
	Weight						
	Reps						
	Weight						
	Reps						
	Weight						
	Reps						
	Weight						
	Reps						
	Weight						
	Reps						
	Weight						
	Reps						
	Weight						
	Reps						
	Weight						
	Reps						
	Weight						

Cardio

Exercise	Calories	Distance	Time

Water Intake _____

Cooldown _____

Feeling ☆ ☆ ☆ ☆ ☆

Notes

Today's Goal _____   (M) (T) (W) (T) (F) ●S ●S

Muscle Group Focus _____   Weight _____   Date/Time _____

Stretch ◯   Warm-Up _____

Strength Training

Exercise		Set 1	Set 2	Set 3	Set 4	Set 5	Set 6
	Reps						
	Weight						
	Reps						
	Weight						
	Reps						
	Weight						
	Reps						
	Weight						
	Reps						
	Weight						
	Reps						
	Weight						
	Reps						
	Weight						
	Reps						
	Weight						
	Reps						
	Weight						
	Reps						
	Weight						

Cardio

Exercise	Calories	Distance	Time

Water Intake _____

Cooldown _____

Feeling ☆ ☆ ☆ ☆ ☆

Notes

Today's Goal _____   (M) (T) (W) (T) (F) **(S) (S)**

Muscle Group Focus _____   Weight _____   Date/Time _____

Stretch ○   Warm-Up _____

Strength Training

Exercise		Set 1	Set 2	Set 3	Set 4	Set 5	Set 6
	Reps						
	Weight						
	Reps						
	Weight						
	Reps						
	Weight						
	Reps						
	Weight						
	Reps						
	Weight						
	Reps						
	Weight						
	Reps						
	Weight						
	Reps						
	Weight						
	Reps						
	Weight						
	Reps						
	Weight						

Cardio

Exercise	Calories	Distance	Time

Water Intake _____

Cooldown _____

Feeling ☆ ☆ ☆ ☆ ☆

Notes

Today's Goal _____   Ⓜ Ⓣ Ⓦ Ⓣ Ⓕ ●S ●S

Muscle Group Focus _____   Weight ____   Date/Time _____

Stretch ○   Warm-Up _____

Strength Training

Exercise		Set 1	Set 2	Set 3	Set 4	Set 5	Set 6
	Reps						
	Weight						
	Reps						
	Weight						
	Reps						
	Weight						
	Reps						
	Weight						
	Reps						
	Weight						
	Reps						
	Weight						
	Reps						
	Weight						
	Reps						
	Weight						
	Reps						
	Weight						
	Reps						
	Weight						

Cardio

Exercise	Calories	Distance	Time

Water Intake _____

Cooldown _____

Feeling ☆ ☆ ☆ ☆ ☆

Notes

Today's Goal _____   (M) (T) (W) (T) (F) **(S) (S)**

Muscle Group Focus _____   Weight _____   Date/Time _____

Stretch ○   Warm-Up _____

Strength Training

Exercise		Set 1	Set 2	Set 3	Set 4	Set 5	Set 6
	Reps						
	Weight						
	Reps						
	Weight						
	Reps						
	Weight						
	Reps						
	Weight						
	Reps						
	Weight						
	Reps						
	Weight						
	Reps						
	Weight						
	Reps						
	Weight						
	Reps						
	Weight						
	Reps						
	Weight						

Cardio

Exercise	Calories	Distance	Time

Water Intake _____

Cooldown _____

Feeling ☆ ☆ ☆ ☆ ☆

Notes

Today's Goal _____   Ⓜ Ⓣ Ⓦ Ⓣ Ⓕ ● ●

Muscle Group Focus _____   Weight _____   Date/Time _____

Stretch ○   Warm-Up _____

Strength Training

Exercise		Set 1	Set 2	Set 3	Set 4	Set 5	Set 6
	Reps						
	Weight						
	Reps						
	Weight						
	Reps						
	Weight						
	Reps						
	Weight						
	Reps						
	Weight						
	Reps						
	Weight						
	Reps						
	Weight						
	Reps						
	Weight						
	Reps						
	Weight						
	Reps						
	Weight						

Cardio

Exercise	Calories	Distance	Time

Water Intake _____

Cooldown _____

Feeling ☆ ☆ ☆ ☆ ☆

Notes

Today's Goal _____   (M) (T) (W) (T) (F) ●S ●S

Muscle Group Focus _____   Weight _____   Date/Time _____

Stretch ○   Warm-Up _____

Strength Training

Exercise		Set 1	Set 2	Set 3	Set 4	Set 5	Set 6
	Reps						
	Weight						
	Reps						
	Weight						
	Reps						
	Weight						
	Reps						
	Weight						
	Reps						
	Weight						
	Reps						
	Weight						
	Reps						
	Weight						
	Reps						
	Weight						
	Reps						
	Weight						
	Reps						
	Weight						

Cardio

Exercise	Calories	Distance	Time

Water Intake _____

Cooldown _____

Feeling ☆ ☆ ☆ ☆ ☆

Notes

Made in the USA
Monee, IL
15 December 2020